Fabiola Méndez Llorente
Jairo Iván Aguilera Soto

Sheep wool

Fabiola Méndez Llorente
Jairo Iván Aguilera Soto

Sheep wool

Production and Quality

ScienciaScripts

Imprint
Any brand names and product names mentioned in this book are subject to trademark, brand or patent protection and are trademarks or registered trademarks of their respective holders. The use of brand names, product names, common names, trade names, product descriptions etc. even without a particular marking in this work is in no way to be construed to mean that such names may be regarded as unrestricted in respect of trademark and brand protection legislation and could thus be used by anyone.

Cover image: www.ingimage.com

This book is a translation from the original published under ISBN 978-620-0-02079-6.

Publisher:
Sciencia Scripts
is a trademark of
Dodo Books Indian Ocean Ltd. and OmniScriptum S.R.L publishing group

120 High Road, East Finchley, London, N2 9ED, United Kingdom
Str. Armeneasca 28/1, office 1, Chisinau MD-2012, Republic of Moldova, Europe
Managing Directors: Ieva Konstantinova, Victoria Ursu
info@omniscriptum.com

Printed at: see last page
ISBN: 978-620-6-76305-5

Sheep wool

Production and quality

Dr. en C. Fabiola Méndez Llorente

Dr. en C. Jairo Iván Aguilera Soto

Content

INTRODUCTION

Sheep is an animal species that has accompanied humans since ancient times, representing a source of food and sustenance (Orona *et al.*, 2014). It presents outstanding characteristics of hardiness, resistance and adaptability, being an excellent option for its development in arid zones (Tinoco, 2009). It is beneficial for the economy, especially for low-income farmers, and due to the high demand for its meat, milk, hides and wool products, especially among the urban population (SAGARPA, 2015). Wool is a natural fiber with unique qualities and characteristics; according to Arrebola *et al.* (2004), it has been the fundamental basis for the production of fabrics since ancient times; it can be processed in an industrial or artisanal manner, and in addition to the manufacture of textiles, it is an excellent option for use in the construction sector.

Although sheep farming is an important activity within livestock production, it is primarily oriented towards meat production, and wool production is insignificant and in many cases represents losses for the owner of the animals. On occasions, sheep are only seen as a simple saving for emergency economic situations, and have given rise to crossbreeding with hair sheep breeds, resulting in the production of low quality wool with coarse fibers. The low value of the wool product has led sheep farmers to consider the advantage of substituting wool breeds to avoid shearing the animals (SAGARPA, 2015).

Since Zacatecas is a nationally recognized entity in the production of sheep wool and due to the little existing information about the macroscopic and microscopic characteristics that it presents, the objective of this work was to collaborate in the study of the characterization of sheep wool fiber, to determine the wool quality in the entity and in this way, take advantage of the best annual production and also, that the sheep farming in the entity is sustainable by preserving the quality of the wool livestock that it presents.

Textile fibers

For years, man has employed the use of animal and vegetable fibers for the elaboration of garments, being these a source of protection to cover his body from the sun, cold and rain (Falconí, 2013).

Fiber is the name given to each of the filaments that, arranged in bundles, are the component of yarns and fabrics of vegetable, animal, mineral or artificial origin (Textile, 2008). Each fiber is composed of millions of long polymeric molecular chains of defined chemical sequence, which are repeated throughout its length, being this number of repetition units, which gives it its degree of polymerization. The fiber is the fundamental unit of textiles (Lockuán, 2013).

Textile fiber is that material that after being subjected to physical and/or chemical processes, yarns are obtained with which fabrics and finally garments are manufactured. For a fiber to be considered a textile fiber, it must comply with three main characteristics: flexibility, fineness and length (Villegas and González, 2013); however, Lockuán (2013) mentions that the three characteristics required must be: flexibility, elasticity and resistance.

Classification of textile fibers

Textile fibers can be classified according to their origin, length and composition (Andrade, 2017).

ASTM Standard D-2368-71 (1975), mentions that fibers for textile use are classified into two major groups: manufactured fibers and fibers of natural origin (Zenteno, 2015).

Fibers of natural origin

Fibers of natural origin are divided into three main groups: vegetable, animal and mineral (Andrade, 2017). They are found in nature and are extracted through chemical and natural processes (Lockuán, 2013).

Around 35 million tons of natural fibers are produced annually from plants and animals, being the livelihood of hundreds of millions of people worldwide (FAO, 2009; Villegas, 2013).

Natural fibers of animal origin

Described by Delgado (2003), natural fibers of animal origin are divided into two main groups: filaments such as silk, and fine hairs. Fine hairs originate from animal hair follicles, and in turn, are divided into two branches: the first of fine fibers or commonly called "special or noble fibers", and the other of wool.

Special or noble fibers

Special or noble fibers are obtained from the hair of goats, various members of the camelid family, rabbits and bovines, the main attraction of these fibers being their softness, luster and fineness. An important aspect that reinforces the exclusivity of these fibers is their scarcity and, therefore, the high prices in relation to other fibers of animal origin. Among the characteristics that make them different from wool are their smaller diameter, low presence of undulations, greater luster and softness.

Lana

By definition, according to ISO 6938-1984, wool consists solely of fibers from sheep breeds (*Ovies aries*).

Grossman (2009) states that wool is considered the "Queen of Fibers", since its natural properties and aptitudes, despite man's attempts, have not been matched.

Sheep species

Sheep are animals that were domesticated more than 7000 years ago (Alvarado, 2018). They have a calm temperament and a gregarious instinct, which is a great advantage in their management (Espinal *et al.*, 2006). They represent the group of animals called small ruminants (FAO, 2019).

The breeding and utilization of this species by humans is known as sheep farming. It is widely distributed throughout the world, being found in a great variety of climates and ecologies (Atto, 2007).

Current situation of sheep farming

In 2017, FAOSTAT statistics reported that the world sheep population reached a total of 1,363,781,956 head, with China, Australia, India, Nigeria, Sudan, Iran and the United Kingdom as the main producers worldwide, with Mexico in 39th place at the continental level. Asia and Europe account for more than 50% of the total sheep population, with the American continent representing 5.9% of this total, with more than 81 million head. In the case of the Americas, the country with the largest number of sheep is Brazil, followed by Argentina and Peru, with Mexico in fourth position (see Table 1). (FAOSTAT, 2020).

Table1 . Countries with the highest sheep production in the Americas

Countries	Heads
Brazil	17,976,367
Argentina	14,842,957
Peru	11,000,424
Mexico	8,902,451
Bolivia	7,442,000
Uruguay	6,565,000
United States	5,250,000
Chile	2,037,516
Cuba	1,567,200
Colombia	1,026,340

Source: FAOSTAT, 2020.

According to reports from SIAP-SAGARPA (2018), the national sheep inventory is estimated at 8,902,451 head, with most of the stock concentrated in the states of Mexico, Hidalgo and Veracruz. Zacatecas ranks sixth with 427,080 head, representing 4.7% of the national herd.

The municipalities with the largest number of sheep in the state of Zacatecas are: Pinos, Sombrerete, Fresnillo and Río Grande (INEGI, 2007). Pinos, the municipality with the largest sheep inventory, has 70,913 head, representing 16.6% at the state level; more sheep stock is reported in this municipality than in states such as Baja California, Baja California Sur, Colima, Morelos, Nayarit, Quintana Roo and Tabasco, representing 0.79% of the national total (Carrera and Carrera, 2011).

Sheep products and by-products

Sheep are one of the animals that humans raise mainly for wool, meat, milk and skins (FAO, 2020).

Wool production

Wool is a fiber formed in the follicles of the sheep skin, which together make up the fleece that covers the body of the whole animal. It is soft, curly and forms part of the variety of natural fibers that contribute to the development of textiles and clothing (Tinoco, 2009).

Wool is a product whose use began in prehistoric times (Gómez, 2017). At the beginning of the last century, only natural fibers such as cotton and wool existed for textile use, sharing their participation in 80 and 20% respectively; then artificial fibers of natural polymers such as rayon, acetate, among others, emerged. It was in the 1970s when a strong substitution of natural fibers for synthetic fibers derived from petroleum began to be imposed, maintaining this trend until the present, where natural fibers represent less than 35% of the total (Mario, 2015). According to Alvarado (2018), worldwide wool represents only 1.6% of natural fibers for textile use.

Statistics from FAOSTAT (2020) show that in 2013, the world production of soiled wool was 2,175,898 tons, with the main producing countries being : China, Australia and New Zealand, which together account for 45% of the total. Mexico ranks 49th in the world. The American continent represents 6.7% of world production with 147,118 tons, with Argentina, Uruguay and the United States being the main producing countries; Mexico is in eighth place.

According to SIAP (2020), in 2018 Mexico obtained 4,530 tons of wool, with 12 Mexican states producing wool. Hidalgo is the main producing state with 45.4%, followed by Zacatecas with 14.1% and the state of Mexico with 11.1%.

Zacatecas has an estimated wool production of 639,666 tons, with Pinos, Ojocaliente, Río Grande, General Francisco R. Murguía and Sombrerete being the main producing municipalities (SIAP, 2018).

Currently, the most widely used Mexican sheep production system is family and extensive. The most widely used sheep breed is Criolla crossed with Rambouillet, Hampshire, Suffolk, Corriedale and Merino sires (Villegas Duran *et al.,* 2001, cited by Peña, 2019).

In the state of Zacatecas, sheep production is carried out in marginalized areas, pasture land and land with agricultural residues, existing as main breeds: Suffolk, Hampshire, Rambouillet and Dorset (Hernández *et al.*, 2017).

Structure of sheepskin

The skin, also known as integument, is one of the largest organs covering the entire surface of the body. Its main function is to act as a natural barrier between the organism and the external environment, providing the necessary protection against physical, chemical and microbiological agents (Costa *et al.*, 2006).

The skin in sheep is thin, flexible and extensible (Pacsi, 2016), presenting thickness measurements of 1 to 3 mm (SPH, 2015).

It is composed of three layers, a more superficial one called epidermis, followed by the dermis and more internally the hypodermis or endodermis (Taipe, 2012).

The epidermis is of a polystratified nature, and the thickness in sheep species varies according to the regions of the body, being thinner in places covered by wool (Costa *et al.,* 2006).

The dermis is the intermediate layer of the skin, it is formed by two layers: one of them is the papillary or thermostatic layer, which includes the hair follicles, sebaceous and sweat glands; and the other is the erector muscle of the hair and the reticular layer (Costa *et al.,* 2006). It is flexible, fibrous, retractile, very resistant and constitutes the main thickness of the skin (Chancusig, 2011).

The endodermis is the part of the skin that ensures the union with the animal's body. It is a lax connective tissue made up of large lobules of fatty tissue limited by partitions of thin collagen fibers and scarce elastic fibers. It is the part corresponding to the adipose tissue and is located under the dermis (Chancusig, 2011).

Follicle structure

The follicle originates from the skin, and divides vertically into several zones. One is called the bulb, extending to the tip of the dermal papilla, where active cell division takes place and fiber formation begins. Another, called the keratogenic zone, which extends upwards from the follicle at the tip of the papilla, where active protein synthesis and cell elongation take place; above this region, the final keratinization (hardening) of the fiber occurs and the degradation of the inner root begins. Finally, there is a detachment zone, where the degraded inner root sheath cells and some cells of the outer root pulp, are introduced into the fiber canal (SPH, 2015).

Accessory structures of the follicle

The follicle is surrounded by sebaceous glands, sweat glands and the erector pili muscle (Elvira, 2009).

The sebaceous glands present a cluster structure constituted by two lobes. They carry out a holocrine secretion, where the final product is of a lipidic nature, formed by a mixture of sterols with fatty acids that chemically constitutes a wax that lubricates the fiber during its growth. Its function is to prevent felting and acts as a water repellent (Galicer, 2015).

Sweat glands have the shape of an unbranched tube. They are made up of cubic-shaped secretory cells, and their ducts lead to shallow depressions located on the cutaneous ridges. Their function is regulated by a neuro-hormonal mechanism, which produces the product suintin, which is composed of water, chlorides, urea, ammonia, ammonia, phosphates and potassium salts of various fatty acids. The main function of sweat is to protect the fiber from ultraviolet rays and also plays an important role in the mechanism of thermoregulation and elimination of toxins (Galicer, 2015).

The secretions of the sebaceous and sweat glands, together with the epithelial desquamations, constitute the so-called suarda. The main function of grease or suarda is to keep the skin lubricated and protect the fiber from the action of external agents. The highest concentration of this grease is found in the upper region of the fleece. When the wool has enough grease or suarda and at the same time it is found uniformly throughout the fiber, we speak of a better quality wool (Falconí, 2013).

The erector pili muscle is formed by bundles of smooth muscle fibers, it is attached at one end to the follicle and at the other to the epidermis. When it contracts, it produces the erection of the hair or wool. In sheep, this muscle is not associated with all hair follicles, and in wool producing breeds, it is not associated with the sweat glands or the so-called secondary follicles (Costa *et al.,* 2006; Badajos, 2007).

The fiber is surrounded by a tubular structure called hair follicle, which covers almost the entire thickness of the dermis (Araoz, 2008).

In sheep skin, there is the presence of primary and secondary hair follicles (Costa *et al.,* 2006).

Primary and secondary follicles

In sheep, there are two types of follicles known as primary and secondary.

Primary follicles develop in the sheep skin during uterine life and begin to produce fibers before birth. They are larger than secondary follicles and therefore tend to develop thicker and longer fibers (medullated fibers and hairs). At birth the population of primary follicles is complete, and their number remains constant throughout life. Primary follicles are approximately 1 mm long, generally shorter in fine wool producing breeds, while in coarse wool producing animals they are longer. Primary follicles are also characterized by being prone to produce fibers with internal air channels, known as medullated fibers. They have an associated sebaceous gland, a sweat gland, and an erector muscle (Elvira, 2009).

Primary follicles are divided into central and lateral, usually arranged in rows on the skin in groups of three, known as trios (SPH, 2015).

Secondary follicles are mainly responsible for wool production. Their size is smaller and they are much more abundant than primary follicles. They have only a sebaceous gland associated with their structure, lacking a sweat gland and erector muscle. Only a part of secondary follicles develop fiber before birth, their maturation is after parturition and adverse conditions in this period can limit the number of secondary follicles and therefore the production of wool. They have the ability to form "bouquets; which are a set of associated follicles where several fibers grow and come to the surface through a single pore of the skin. The number of secondary follicles in sheep skin is higher in those breeds that produce finer wool (Elvira, 2009).

Follicular density

Follicular density is the number of fibers per unit area. When the sheep is born, the hair follicles are compacted in the skin, generally presenting a high density; as the animal grows and the skin expands, the follicular density decreases. Density is an interesting characteristic for the producer, since the higher the density, the greater the fleece weight (Araoz, 2008).

Primary/secondary follicular ratio

The ratio of secondary to primary follicles, is a useful indicator of the quality (density and fineness) of wool fiber production in sheep. It is commonly referred to as the S/P ratio (SPH, 2015).

The number of primary follicles is similar for all breeds, while the number of secondary follicles varies, thus determining the different S/P ratios of each breed. This is ratio is not constant among sheep breeds (Elvira, 2009; SPH, 2015).

Follicles are found in follicular groups, formed by the primary trio surrounded by several associated secondary follicles, thus being the basic unit of wool production (Araoz, 2008; SPH, 2015;).

Biological development of wool fiber (physiology)

The growth of a wool fiber, is a dynamic process in which cell multiplication and migration takes place, along with the biosynthesis of a complex mixture of proteins that form the fiber and internal root (SPH, 2015).

Fiber growth begins in the papilla, which is an invagination or internal folding of skin cells within the follicle. These cells have the ability to actively multiply (grow and divide). The new cells resulting from the division are expelled through the follicle channel by further multiplication, generating a constant flow of cells to the skin surface. Before emerging on the surface, the columnar cells pass through a hardening zone located in the first third of the length of the follicle. There, chemical bonds occur in a process called keratinization, causing changes in the cellular protein from a soft to a "hard" keratinized protein. When the process of wool production is complete, the fibrous material emerging from the skin surface is dead tissue, similar in chemical structure to hair, nails, claws, hooves, horns and feathers (Araoz, 2008; Elvira, 2009;).

Types of fiber produced by sheep

Adult sheep produce three main types of fibers: true wool fibers, med fibers and kemp fibers. True wool fibers can grow from both primary and secondary follicles, depending on the breeding. Kemp and med fibers grow only from primary follicles (SPH, 2015).

Med fibers

Med (pile, or heterotype) fibers are medullated, meaning that they have air channels within them and tend to be finer than kemp fibers. Med fibers are generally as long as "true" wool fibers but may lack crimp. These fibers are very difficult to detect with the naked eye (SPH, 2015).

Kemp fibers

Kemp are the coarsest fibers that grow on sheep, and usually shed seasonally. Kemps tend to be short, chalky, white, brittle, and do not seem to accept dyes well. Kemp fiber is hard to handle and is undesirable (SPH, 2015).

Wool fibers

True wool fibers, is the commercial product associated with the sheep industry (SPH, 2015).

Wool fiber structure

Wool fiber has a curly and wavy structure, with an apparent length, which changes when extended. It is resistant, elastic and flexible (Tinoco, 2009).

Toapanta (2016) mentions that the typical color of wool is white, but it can vary from black, gray, brown or more shades.

The main distinguishing characteristics of wool are its lack of medullation and the presence of crimp with varying degrees of crimp (SPH, 2015).

Internal wool fiber morphology

The wool fiber is composed of three prototypes of cells: the first, which covers the fiber in the form of scaly cell layers or cuticle, the second, which is found underneath it forming the body of the fiber or cortex, and the third, the medullar cells, in case there is a pith forming a channel in the central axis of the fiber (Delgado, 2003).

Cuticle

The cuticle is the outer layer of the fiber composed of flat epithelial cells, which longitudinally and peripherally slightly overlap each other forming a protective layer of cells called scales (Arrebola *et al.,* 2004).

The scales are rarely found in more than two layers, and thanks to them, it is possible to identify the woolly fiber from other animal hairs and the rest of the textile fibers. They provide the fiber with particular strength and during growth, they keep it fastened within the follicle. They give the fiber many of its excellent characteristics (SPH, 2015).

The cuticle protects the fiber from mechanical damage and climatic influences (Delgado, 2003).

Each cuticular cell is composed of three layers called: exocuticle, endocuticle and epicuticle (Arrebola, 2002).

The epicuticle, which covers the cuticle with a hard and resistant membrane composed of fatty acids, is very resistant to chemical agents and prevents the entry of dyes during the dyeing process; however, it disappears during washing and carding due to its sensitivity to mechanical treatments. The exocuticle and endocuticle are vulnerable to exogenous agents (Arrebola *et al.,* 2004).

Bark

The bark is the main component of wool fiber and constitutes 90% of it (Arrebola, 2002). It imparts the fiber with many special properties including elasticity, strength and durability (SPH, 2015).

It is formed by long, elongated cortical cells arranged parallel to the fiber axis, have a variable size and are aligned like cigarettes (Delgado, 2003).

Within the cortical cells are smaller anatomical units called macrofibrils. Macrofibrils are filamentous bundles, composed of other small units called microfibrils, which are further reduced to structures called protofibrils. Each protofibril contains three helical molecular chains called alpha helices (SPH, 2015).

In the cortex there are different types of cells: orthocortex (orthocortex), paracortex (paracortex) and, in very few cases, mesocortex (mesocortex) (Delgado, 2003). Each cell type has different chemical and physical properties, which are differentiated by their density. The paracortex is located on the inside of the curl curve and the orthocortex on the outside. The relationship between the cortical cells and the crimp, are responsible for the undulations presented by the wool fiber (SPH,2015)

Pigments, according to Delgado (2003), are components present in the cortex, which determine the natural color of the fibers. The colors arise from the accumulation of two types of melanin: eumelanin and pheomelanin. Generally, these are found between the macrofibrils and occasionally in the endocuticle. Natural colors present both types of melanins, but in different compositions and concentrations. While eumelanin produces shades from brown to black, blond and reddish fibers are due to the presence of pheomelanin.

Marrow

It is formed by empty cells (vacuoles) with amorphous protein skeletons and thin filaments. It is a channel located along the central axis of the fiber and originates in the papilla of certain primary follicles. It can be found in a continuous or fragmented form, occupying different proportions of the center of the fiber. Its presence is common in thick fibers (Delgado, 2003).

Medullation is thought to be the result of incomplete keratinization (cornification of the fiber). Basically, the fiber is too wide for the follicle to fill with keratin and a loose or spongy core (SPH, 2015).

Biological composition of sheep wool

According to Romero (2005), sheep wool is biologically composed of fibers (48 to 70%), suard (10 to 25%), water (10 to 20%), internal atmosphere (1%) and aggregates from the external environment such as soil, parasites, fungi, etc. (10 to 20%).

In addition to wool, the fleece contains hairs, which have a different structure with a larger diameter, presence of pith, smooth surface and little elasticity (Falconí, 2013).

Chemical composition of sheep wool fiber

Sheep fiber presents an elemental chemical composition of: Carbon, Hydrogen, Oxygen, Nitrogen and Sulfur, in different percentages (Pesok, 2015).

Table2 . Elemental chemical composition of sheep wool.

Average chemical composition of sheep wool					
Element	C	H	O	N	S
%	50	7	22-25	16-17	3-4

Source: Rosas, 2016.

The main component of wool is keratin, which is the result of a polymerization of amino acids with high sulfur content (Fernández *et al.,* 2012). There are 19 different amino acids combined and united in polypeptide chains folded on themselves, in such a way that they act like spiral springs. This internal elasticity added to the extensibility of the external crimp of the fiber, give it a continuous stretching potential, which explains the great elasticity and natural resistance of wool (SPH, 2015).

The relative amount of amino acids can vary from sample to sample, for different areas of the same fleece (Pesok, 2015). The main molecular chains of wool keratin, linked by cystine or sulfur cross-links and salt bridges, are capable of assuming two different configurations, depending on whether or not the fiber is in a stressed state. Alpha (α) keratin refers to the molecule in its relaxed state, while beta (β) keratin in designating the molecule in the stretched state. Keratin beta is analogous to other fiber molecules, while the alpha type is associated exclusively with wool.

There is no chemical difference between the two types. It is a property of beta keratin to resume the alpha form when stress is removed from the fiber. Therefore, the mechanism of the unusual elasticity of wool fiber is that of a molecular spring (SPH, 2015).

Table3 . Average composition of amino acids present in sheep wool.

Amino acid	%
Alanine	4.12
Arginine	19.10
Aspartic acid	4.38
Cystine	7.30
Glutamic Acid	8.48
Glycine	6.49
Histidine	1.91
Isoleucine	2.44
Lysine	3.92
Methionine	0.32
Phenylalin	2.12
Valina	4.16
Serina	8.66
Threonine	5.12
Tryptophan	0.82
Leucine	5.85

Source: Pesok, 2015.

Methods for obtaining sheep wool

During the year, sheep wool presents a constant growth and tends to shed naturally in an attempt to acclimatize for the new season, however, there are some breeds that do not lose wool naturally. With excess wool, sheep can accumulate dirt, excrement, insect pests, fleas, ticks, as well as fungi in damp areas and other particles that affect fleece quality. In order to preserve the welfare and health of the animal, sheep should be sheared once a year (Rosas, 2016).

Shearing

The task of separating the fleece from the animal by shearing is called shearing. Although it is generally done once a year, some producers do it twice a year (Romero, 2005).

The purpose of shearing is to obtain the wool that has been growing, presenting advantages such as the productive use of the wool, improving animal welfare, mitigating the effects of heat in summer and allowing the animal to move easily (Martínez *et al.*, 2019).

Shearing during the spring, allows the sheep to have short and clean wool during the summer, improving its quality (Rosas, 2016).

Shearing can be done manually with the use of appropriate scissors, or mechanically by employing two-bladed machines that operate using electric motive power (Toapanta, 2016).

There are two shearing techniques used in different parts of the world according to local traditions: the Creole or "maneado" method and the "tally hi", "tally hi" or Australian method. In the "maneado" method, the animal is tied before the fleece is cut, being the most traditional and oldest technique. The Australian method is performed without tethering by positioning the animal in a seated position (Toapanta, 2016).

Sheep, regardless of breed, can produce between 2.3 and 3.6 kg of gross wool per year, 1 to 3 kg of fine wool, and 2 to 3 kg of coarse wool depending on the fleece (Rosas, 2016; SIAP, 2018).

Classification of sheep wool

According to Falconí (2013), in ancient times, wool was classified according to the area of the animal's body where it came from; however, today it is considered too much work and is not economically justified.

Table4 . Fleece characteristics in sheep according to body region.

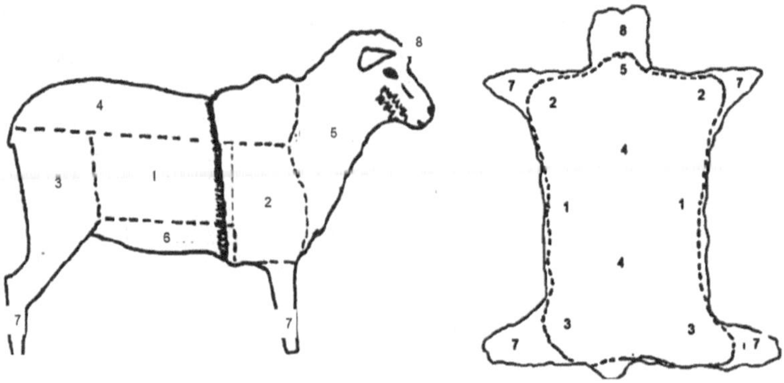

Regions (parts of the fleece)	Description
1 Rib	The most representative, of superior quality.
2 Palette	The finest. Long and uniform strands. Standard zone for comparison with other zones.
3 Quarts	Wool thicker than the rest, not uniform, prone to be medullated, contain seed and pilling.
4 Loin	Most affected by climate action, prone to be contaminated.
5 Chest	Good wool, somewhat less regular.
6 Belly	Wool of regular quality, shorter, and often contaminated with urine and vegetable matter.
7 Claws	Short, coarse, medullated, contaminated and rough wool, containing hairs and little wool. For use in low quality manufacturing and blending with other wools.
8 Head	Short, coarse, medullated, contaminated, coarse wool containing hairs.

Source: Guzman, 2009; Alvarado, 2018.

Wool fiber is highly variable; it is not a uniform biological product. In addition to being produced by different breeds, all with different characteristics, even within the same breed and in the same environment, no two fleeces are exactly alike (Romero, 2005). This is due to the different skin structures, as well as the nature of the wool-producing follicles in the different regions of the body (Arrebola *et al.,* 2004).

Once the wool is obtained, it is classified according to the criteria of fineness, length, strength and yield (Tinoco, 2009; Toapanta, 2016).

It must be characterized, highlighting its qualitative and quantitative attributes, especially if it is presumed to be heterogeneous, so that its quality can be identified (Gómez, 2017). Each country manages its own grading standard, however, in international trade micronage is used as an objective measure (Romero, 2005).

Martinez *et al.* (2019), mention that in practice wool is classified as: super fine or fine, intermediate, coarse and very coarse.

Super fine or fine wool

This wool has a diameter < 20.9 microns.

Intermediate wool

It measures from 21 to 29.9 microns.

Coarse wool

This wool is between 30 and 36.9 microns in diameter.

Wool very thick

This type of wool has diameters >37 microns.

Characteristics of wool

Diameter

The diameter is the thickness or fineness measured in microns (μ); that is, it is the measurement of the cross section of the wool fiber (Lobos and Pavez, 2018). The most representative area to evaluate the diameter is in the middle rib of the animal (Guzmán, 2009).

Since it is a constant variable among breeds, it contributes to their differentiation (Toapanta, 2016). It can have a variation from 10 to 70 microns, being of higher price those with lower thickness (Lobos and Pavez, 2018).

Diameter is directly related to wool fineness (Saldaña, 2017), and is most important measurement for fiber classification, which can determine its price in the market (Araoz, 2019).

The average diameter, results from the average of the diameter of the clean wool fibers and is the commercial characteristic of greatest importance; as for the coefficient of variation, it is the comparison of the variations in fiber diameter between wools with different diameter values (Gómez, 2017).

Length

Length is the distance between the base and the tip of the wool fiber expressed in cm (Lobos and Pavez, 2018). It refers to the measurement in a natural way, in a year of growth, which, due to their natural origin, present a variable measurement (Araoz, 2019).

Two types are obtained: relative length, referring to the length of the strand measured from the root to the tip, determined without stretching the natural crimps; and absolute length, obtained by making the fiber crimps disappear (Toapanta, 2016). The relationship between them is called elongation ratio (Arrebola *et al*, 2004).

It is the second characteristic in order of importance (Zúñiga, 2011), which, like diameter, constitutes one of the most important parameters for classification and determination of subsequent use in the textile process (Araoz, 2019).

Fleece weight

The fleece weight is obtained after shearing (Araoz, 2019). It is represented in kg and both the weight of dirty fleece and the weight of clean fleece are obtained after having been subjected to washing and drying (Toapanta, 2016).

Performance

It is the ratio of the weight of the clean fleece to the weight of the dirty fleece after washing (Sabina, 2019). Since wool usually contains fats and impurities, the yield informs about the total amount of fiber available. It is expressed in RINDO units, equivalent to percent yield (Saldaña, 2017).

Undulations and character

Ripples in wool fiber are curves or waves that have as their fundamental principles regular, successive and uniform curves, placed in the same plane along the entire fiber (Lobos and Pavez, 2018).

The shape and number of crimps is a hereditary character. When a fleece has well marked waviness, with uniform curves from the base to the tip, it represents a quality index and is what is called "Character", which is the third characteristic, in importance, for the qualitative appreciation of the fleece (Toapanta, 2016).

Wool fiber crimps are quantified in crimp frequency/cm (Gomez, 2017).

Curvature index

Curl is a natural undulation, which produces the force for fiber swelling and elasticity. The degree of curvature is associated with crimp or crimp of the strands and is measured in degrees per millimeter (Lobos and Pavez, 2018). Thus, the fiber with the highest degree of curl per millimeter has the highest number of crimps. The curl with lower degree to 50 degrees/mm, is described as low curl; the curl with a range of 60 to 90 degrees/mm is considered as medium curl, and high curl, are those greater than 100 degrees/mm (Guzman, 2009).

The bending of the fibers can be in three dimensions, because the fibers are bent and twisted along their entire length. However, because most of the bending occurs in one plane and bending has the largest contribution, the fiber shape can be represented in a two-dimensional waveform (Quispe *et al.,* 2013).

Color

Wool has a slightly yellowish white color, and there are also dark wools (black or brown) due to the melanin content; these wools are used in the production of products that do not have to undergo dyeing processes (Cazares, 2011). Dark fiber is considered to be that which departs from the white color with a degree of coloration greater than 5, on a scale of 0 to 8 (Sánchez, 2010).

Pigmented wools are a minority and particular production within the sheep wool production, however, it is a product in increasing valuation by the market of handmade products and as such, it exhibits important prices (Lobos and Pavez, 2018).

The wool's own characteristics are identical in both variants and their only difference is their color (Sabina, 2019).

Brightness

Ideally, wool should be white and bright (Botha and Hunter, 2010). Toapanta (2016) mentions that the luster, is due to the reflection of light on the free part of the cuticular cells of the fiber, offering different degrees. The Silver Luster, which occurs in fine and wavy fibers (Merino), because the smaller scales offer little surface and many free edges that refract light and give a white matte dye. The Silk Luster, which occurs in thick and long wools (Lincoln), because the cuticle cells are less overlapped and offer a greater reflection giving it a remarkable brightness. And Glassy Luster, which occurs in the case of Angora goat hair.

In the Australian method, brightness in wool is referred to in terms of L *, and yellowness in terms of b *, while in the New Zealand method Y and Y - Z were used, respectively. Y indicates the brightness (whiteness) of the wool, the higher the value of Y, the better the brightness of the wool, and the lower the yellowness (Y - Z) the better. However, the IWTO in 1997 recommended implementing the measurement system with a 10º observation angle and D65 illumination system (D65 / 10º), the official change occurred in 2002, where L* (brightness) would correspond to Y, and a* corresponding to Y - Z (yellowness) (Botha and Hunter, 2010).

Density

The density of wool is given by the number of fibers in a given area of skin, expressed in cm^2 or square inch. The amount of wool produced and thus the weight of the fleece will depend on this (Toapanta, 2016).

Comfort

The comfort factor is referred to as the threshold level indicator of comfort in wool (Gomez, 2017). It is provided by fibers smaller than 30 microns. Itchiness in fabrics is due to the fineness of the ends of coarse fibers which, being less flexible, protrude from the surface of the yarns. However, if the end of those fibers are thinner and therefore more flexible, they are less likely to cause itching (Lobos and Pavez, 2018).

Properties of sheep wool

The properties of sheep wool allow us to know the behavior of the fiber and, in addition, the possibilities of its utilization and final use (Andrade, 2017).

Chemical properties

Action of acids, bases and solvents

Wool fiber is composed of many amino acids, some of which are acidic and some of which are basic (SPH, 2015).

It is resistant to the action of mild or diluted acids, but on the other hand, concentrated mineral acids such as sulfuric and nitric acids cause fiber splitting and decomposition (Zúñiga, 2011).

Alkalis act mainly on the keratin of the fiber, hydrolyzing the polypeptide chain, attacking some amino acid remainder and creating new transverse bonds. When wool is attacked by alkalis there is a loss of resistance, its color tends to be yellowish, the touch is rougher, affecting its commercial quality (Saldaña, 2017). Sodium hydroxide solutions at 5%, at room temperature, dissolve the wool fiber (Zúñiga, 2011).

Organic solvents commonly used to clean and remove stains from wool fabrics do not damage wool fibers (Chancusig, 2011).

Water action

The ionic bonds of acidic, basic and hydrogen amino acids contribute to stabilize the structure of dry keratin. Both bonds are broken as the keratin absorbs water, which can be up to 34% of its dry weight. Wool becomes more susceptible to chemical damage in aqueous media because the protein chains can be ionized and attract small molecules of acids and alkalis. Wools well washed in a weak alkaline medium, do not produce a significant alteration of the fiber, since they should have an aqueous extract pH between 9 and 10 and the temperature should not be higher than 50ºC (Saldaña, 2017).

Chlorine effect

When wool comes into contact with chlorine, it makes it hard and brittle, causing the loss of its weight, elasticity and filtering power. However, it improves its brightness and affinity to dyes (Cazares, 2008).

Physical properties

Hygroscopicity

Hygroscopicity is defined as the ability of textile fibers to absorb water from the atmosphere, retain it and remove it (Saldaña, 2017). Wool fiber is the most hygroscopic of the textile fibers, varying according to relative humidity (SPH, 2015).

Rosas (2016) mentions that wool has an absorption capacity of up to 50% without producing runoff, varying according to the temperature and humidity in which it is found. This capacity of the fiber contributes to the comfort of wool-based garments (SPH, 2015).

Extensibility or elongation

This property allows the wool fiber to stretch in great proportion, increasing its length by up to 30% (Zúñiga, 2011); this is due to its histological structure and the absence of pith (Flores, 2012).

This is considered important from the textile point of view, since industrialization processes such as carding, combing and spinning subject the fibers to considerable stresses, which must have sufficient extensibility to remain intact during these processes (Chancusig, 2011).

Extensibility is determined by means of the dynamometer, stretching the fiber to the "breaking point" which is expressed as a percentage of its original length or in millimeters per 10 cm (Flores, 2012).

Elasticity

This property is directly related to elongation, since after the fiber increases its size, it has the ability to recover its natural state in 99%, due to the helical structure in its molecules. Thanks to this extension recovery property, wool has the ability to retain the shape of the garments and maintain the elasticity of the yarns (Zúñiga, 2011).

Fine wools are more elastic than coarse wools (Arrebola *et al.*, 2004).

Resistance

Strength is the tensile stress that a wool fiber is able to withstand before breaking (Toapanta, 2016).

Not all the fibers of the sheep's body have the same resistance, this will depend on the area of the animal's body, for example, those found in the back present greater resistance than those found in the abdomen (Mueller and Cueto, 2010).

Fiber strength is measured in units of Newtons/kilotex (N/ktex), recording values in the range of 2 to 100 (SPH, 2015).

Flexibility

It is the property presented by the wool fiber, with which it can be easily bent without cracking or breaking (Toapanta, 2016). This is of great importance for the industry, both in spinning and weaving, to obtain resistant fabrics (Chancusig, 2011).

Because of this, products and garments made from wool do not wrinkle easily (Cazares, 2008).

Breathability

Wool is a fiber that has an active response to fluctuations in body temperature. When worn as a garment, it allows the skin to breathe easily. Wool has the natural ability to transpire and absorb up to 35% of its weight in water (moisture) due to its hydrophilic core. This moisture is then naturally released as vapor into the air, causing adequate comfort. No other fiber offers this property (Mueller and Cueto, 2010).

Infiltration

It is an intrinsic and unique property of wool, considered as the capacity of the fibers to form a compact mass impossible to unravel, depending on the length, fineness, crimp and external scaly structure of the fiber. The larger the diameter of the fiber, the lower its felting capacity (Cazares, 2008).

Temperature effects

When wool is exposed to moderately low temperatures there is no effect, however, at extremely low temperatures (liquid nitrogen), the fiber becomes very brittle. When fibers are exposed to ultraviolet rays in sunlight, a photochemical reaction occurs in the disulfide bond and other parts of the keratin molecule, expressed by a yellowing of the exposed wool tips. This explains the "frowzy" and "eroded" tips of some fibers that have little grease to filter the sun's ultraviolet rays. When wool exceeds 100°C for some time, it decomposes, and acquires a yellow color that eventually turns brown. On the other hand, if it is heated to less than 100ºC it becomes rough, recovering its soft feel when it retains moisture (SPH, 2015).

Action on fire

Unlike other fibers, wool is not flammable, since its high water and nitrogen content make it a fire retardant, complying with many international regulations without the need for chemical treatments (Mueller and Cueto, 2010). As it does not support combustion, in case of contact with fire it reacts with low propagation and little smoke production, and in case of fire it will be extinguished (Rosas, 2016).

Although wool fibers are self-extinguishing, they can burn only with a very intense heat source and abundant oxygen supply (SPH, 2015).

Thermal qualities

Wool is an excellent thermal insulator, this due to its curling, volume and resistance qualities, which allow at the time of fabric processing, to form trapped air spaces that result in its insulating capacity against both high and low temperatures (Molina, 2013; SPH, 2015).

It provides warmth and shelter in cold weather generating a temperate effect, and is self-adapting when the temperature rises releasing heat and moisture to maintain a comfortable and cool climate (Mueller and Cueto, 2010).

Abrasion resistance

It is defined as the fiber's capacity to withstand rubbing or fiction. It is an important property in wool applications, but above all, in those for making rugs, carpets, linings and ropes (Andrade, 2017).

Tensile strength

During textile processing, wool fibers are subjected to various tractions that can achieve breakage. Tensile strength can be described as the tensile force required to break a known amount of wool or fiber. It is measured in Newton/kilotex, where Newton is a force or load and kilotex is the linear density of a strand (Quispe *et al.*, 2013).

Acoustic property

Sheep wool has acoustic properties, therefore, it absorbs and reduces noise levels (Rosas, 2016).

Durability.

Wool is a long-lived material, its durability condition implies maintaining its moisture retention and flexibility properties without losing its structure and elasticity when properly cared for. This has been exemplified historically by carpets, which can withstand intensive use without losing their appearance (Mueller and Cueto, 2010).

Biodegradable action

Sheep wool can absorb and decompose pollutants (formaldehyde, nitrogen dioxide and sulfur dioxide) from indoor air, thus improving its quality. All this decreases the impact with the environment (Rosas, 2016).

It can biodegrade in soil without any harm to the environment, meeting optimal product life cycle requirements (Mueller and Cueto, 2010).

Biological properties

Sheep wool has a certain resistance to microorganisms such as bacteria and fungi, however, if stored in the presence of moisture and dust, they generate rotting that can destroy the fiber. However, these microorganisms attack the stains that appear on the wool (Toapanta, 2016).

Factors affecting sheep wool quality and quantity

There are different factors in sheep such as gestation, lactation, sex, age, health and climate, which can influence wool production. All these factors act on the daily fiber production in the follicles and, therefore, influence wool characteristics such as fleece weight, length, diameter, resistance, among others (Quispe *et al.,* 2013).

Genetic influences

Many fiber and follicle characteristics are highly heritable. The maximum rate of wool or hair production in a sheep and the range of variation in quality-related characteristics is established by its genotype. There are definite differences among sheep breeds in production capacity and fleece characteristics. Similarly, within breeds and individually there is considerable variation in wool growth rate (Khan *et al.*, 2012).

Physiological and environmental influences

Effects during fetal and early postnatal life.

During the period when the follicle is developing, it can be adversely affected by inadequate nutrient supply. Poor feeding of the ewe during the last third of gestation, when the demand for nutrients for fetal growth is greatest, as well as of the lamb during the first months of life, may prevent or delay the development of some follicles. Maturation of secondary follicles may be delayed up to 6 to 12 months, or the capacity for fiber production may be permanently impaired (Khan *et al.*, 2012).

Adult wool production is lower in sheep born and reared as twins, and in sheep born to young ewes. These disadvantages generally equate to a reduction in annual clean fleece weight of 0.1 to 0.2 kg, and are likely related to restricted nutrient supply in utero and during early lactation (Khan *et al.*, 2012).

Effects during adulthood

The amount and type of fiber produced in the adult stage is influenced by a variety of physiological and environmental factors (Khan *et al.*, 2012).

Nutrition

In sheep, feeding plays an important role in follicle formation and maturation, as well as in fiber growth and diameter. Thus, in periods of low forage availability, fiber diameter is not only reduced, but also fiber production decreases. Wool growth is very sensitive to the levels of energy and protein ingested by the animals (Quispe *et al.,* 2013).

Energy appears to be the main factor in the diet related to wool growth, however, protein supply is also important. A balanced mix of essential amino acids is required, and the addition of sulfur amino acids in the diet plays an important role in regulating wool growth and composition. The main requirement is cystine, but methionine, which can be readily converted to cystine, is equally effective in stimulating wool growth. An increase in cystine supply to the follicles increases the proportion of ultra-high sulfur proteins and thus the sulfur content of wool (Khan *et al.*, 2012).

Minerals such as zinc and copper have shown specific effects on wool fiber growth. A zinc deficiency in sheep produces brittle wool, and an extreme deficiency results in decreased fiber growth and wool shedding (Khan *et al.*, 2012). Copper deficiency produces "steely" or "striped" wool, which lacks curl and has a shiny or silky appearance, with low strength, elasticity and affinity for dyes, and in severe cases black wool depigmentation. Sulfur deficiency in sheep is unlikely, and if this occurs, it is related to a very deficient protein diet (Martinez *et al.*, 2018).

Age

Young animals tend to produce less wool per unit of feed intake, probably due to competition for nutrients between follicles and other tissues (Khan *et al.*, 2012). Fleece weight is lower than in adults due to body surface area size, however, fibers are finer, as shearing has the effect of increasing follicular functioning. As age increases, fleece weight and diameter increase (Quispe *et al.,* 2013).

Maximum fleece weights in sheep have been observed from three to five years of age, with variable rates of decline in wool production thereafter, as the number of active follicles decreases with age. Several quality characteristics tend to deteriorate and curl abnormalities may appear. These reductions in wool growth with age could be related to changes in feed intake patterns and diet selection (Khan *et al.*, 2012).

Sex

Males tend to produce more wool than females, mainly due to their larger size and better feeding, however, according to Quispe *et al.* (2013) sex does not influence fiber diameter.

Physiological state

The decrease in growth and wool diameter during gestation and lactation have been reported in sheep in stabling and grazing. Pregnant and lactating ewes have fibers with smaller diameter, length and tensile strength (Quispe *et al.,* 2013).

During gestation and early lactation, annual fleece growth in females is generally reduced by 10 to 14%, with the greatest reduction in females rearing twins (Khan *et al.*, 2012). It appears that proteins that escape ruminal degradation in females during the last third of gestation and early lactation are responsible for increasing wool growth, a situation that can be improved when higher protein feeds are introduced in the ration (Quispe *et al.,* 2013).

Nutritional Status

Nutritional status is the result of the balance between energy consumption and expenditure. When the balance is positive, reserves are accumulated in the form of fatty tissue, and if it is negative, these reserves will be consumed. The animal's body reserves are another way of transferring energy obtained from periods of greater availability to periods of scarcity. A large number of factors affect the nutritional status of animals that obtain their main source of food through grazing. A sheep with good nutrition will produce good fleece characteristics (Quispe *et al.*, 2013).

Maternal nutrition influences wool production in the adult life of the lamb. When poor nutrition is present, the follicular S/P ratio is affected in the last third of gestation and first weeks of life. Poor pre-natal nutrition restricts the animal's future ability to produce wool by altering the formation of secondary follicles, and similarly, poor nutrition after birth delays the maturation of these follicles, causing some follicles to never mature. This affects wool production in adult sheep by up to 12% (Martinez *et al.*, 2018).

Hormones

Pituitary hormones including thyroid stimulating hormone, adrenocorticotropic hormone and growth hormone exert a controlling influence on wool growth. Removal of the pituitary gland causes the growth rate to decrease to zero, and thyroidectomy reduces, but does not eliminate wool growth. In both situations, normal wool growth is restored by administration of thyroxine or its active form, triiodothyronine. Adrenocorticotropic hormone causes increased glucocorticoid secretion by the adrenal gland; in sheep, high plasma cortisol concentrations are associated with depression or complete cessation of wool growth (Khan *et al.*, 2012).

Health

The presence of microbial infections and parasites can reduce wool production. All grazing sheep are affected, with the effects being greater at younger ages, causing reductions in wool growth of up to 60% (Khan *et al.*, 2012).

Climate and photoperiod

Climate, with seasonal variations, has an impact on fiber growth and diameter, due to annual rainfall and its effect on forage production (Quispe *et al.,* 2013).

Exposure to heat or cold, or changes in skin temperature, cause a delay in wool growth, especially length due to low temperatures. These effects are related to reduced blood flow and therefore nutrient supply (Khan *et al.*, 2012).

The effects of photoperiod on wool growth have an influence on the cyclic activity of follicles. Seasonal shedding cycles and the annual rhythm of wool growth rate are controlled by day length (Khan *et al.*, 2012).

Pigmented fibers

Sheep wool fibers can be genetically pigmented or stained by feces and urine (Frey, 2007).

Wool pigmentation is a characteristic of primitive sheep. It corresponds to a wool of high thickness, low comfort index, uniformity of diameter, less elasticity, rough to the touch, with different levels of pigmentation and usually accompanied by hairs. The production of this type of wool is highly heritable and is little determined by climatic or nutritional factors. Exceptionally, pigmented wool with good fineness and absence of hair can appear in Merino sheep (Martinez *et al.*, 2018).

Pigmented wools are a minority production, however, it corresponds to a product in increasing valuation by the market for the manufacture of handicraft products and as such, it exhibits important prices in tourist regions (Martínez *et al.*, 2018).

Impurities and contamination

Impurities found in wool can be of natural or acquired origin, generally comprising between 20 and 80% of the total weight of the fiber. Natural impurities are due to the natural secretions of the follicle accessory glands in the sheep's skin, which vary in quantity according to the animal's nutrition. Acquired impurities are foreign matter to the fiber, generally consisting of grass, dust, straw, thistles, stones, excrement and animal urine (Cazares, 2011).

Uses of sheep wool

Textile and handicraft use

The variability of textile fibers produced by sheep currently has two well-defined destinations, industrial and artisanal. The industry manufactures articles and garments for mass consumption, where there is a tendency to select the uniformity of the fibers. In the artisanal activity, garments and fabrics are generally made for family use or for sale to regional tourism, where the aim is to conserve the variability of sheep wool fibers, and the activity also improves the economy of the artisans. In both cases, it is possible to produce a variety of garments such as bags, sweaters, coats, gloves, wallets and a variety of other items, with all kinds of designs and colors (Sabina, 2019).

Thermal insulation

The wool produced by sheep is a biological resource, which can be called a bioproduct. It has shown great potential due to its characteristics and properties that is increasing, being commercialized and gaining space in the market as an alternative insulator (Rosas, 2016). In standard construction, the use of raw materials extracted from nature is employed. The consumption of non-renewable resources and the generation of polluting waste associated with their manufacture and use generate a large amount of environmental impacts. Faced with this problem, the construction sector is undergoing a change in the manufacture of sustainable construction products. This involves the design of products in which the raw materials must be renewable, that is, of natural origin, ensuring the continuity of their renewal. And when the useful life of the material has ended, it can be reintroduced in a new recycling (Wadel, 2009). The manufacture of thermal and acoustic insulation based on sheep wool is less polluting than others and can be done in an artisanal way. Wool has natural properties of temperature regulation, performance, hygroscopicity and fire resistance, which define it as a renewable natural raw material for use as insulation (Rosas, 2016).

Sheep wool in the form of rigid boards is used as thermal and acoustic insulation for floors, walls and roofs in both new constructions and renovation works It is a hygroscopic material that absorbs and releases humidity, maintaining a dry interior environment, and due to the structure of the fiber, it limits the transmission of airborne noise. In combination with other natural materials such as wood, it allows a drastic reduction of the environmental impact, generating an adequate use of wool (Wadel, 2009).

Determination of wool characteristics

Fiber diameter

Fiber diameters can be analyzed on the FibreLux equipment® (Techonology Innovation Agency, South Africa). A small portion of wool sample is taken and manually carded with the help of a brush to parallelize the fibers and remove adhering plant matter. They are placed inside special cartridges and introduced into the equipment, which analyzes the value corresponding to the micronage of each sample.

Fiber length

The length is determined with the help of a ruler graduated in centimeters. The wool fiber is taken and initially the relative length is measured, that is to say, when the fiber was in its natural state (with the undulations without stretching); subsequently, the fiber is stretched and the measurement corresponding to the absolute length is taken, making for each sample the measurement of two individual fibers.

Number of fiber crimps

The wool fiber is placed on a black background, and with the help of a ruler marked in centimeters and a magnifying glass, each of the crimps present per centimeter of fiber is measured. For each sample, two individual fiber crimps are counted.

Brightness

Lightness was obtained with the KONICA MINOLTA ® colorimeter model CHROMA METER CR-400/410. A portion of wool was taken from each of the samples and placed in a cylindrical container. The equipment was introduced into the container of the same circumference, and yielded the values corresponding to the brightness in the fibers, where the variations in lightness (L*) range from white (100) to black (0).

Performance

For the calculation of wool yield, the procedure described by Alata *et al.* (2000) is used, where 5g of each wool sample is weighed on an analytical scale (obtaining the dirty weight), then they are placed inside meshes to proceed to washing, in which the samples are immersed in hot water at 50ºC for 5 minutes, then in hot water with neutral detergent for 5 minutes, shaking the samples simulating the principles of a washing machine. After this, they are introduced in a container with alcohol for 5 minutes, then in hydrogen peroxide for 5 more minutes and then rinsed with common water. Once the samples have been drained, they are removed from the nets and placed in small trays to be taken to a laboratory oven for 60 minutes at 56ºC to dry them. Once the drying time has elapsed, the wool samples are removed from the oven and weighed again on the analytical scale. In this way, the washing yield (difference between the weight of dirty wool and clean wool expressed as a percentage) is obtained.

Humidity

The FibreLux equipment ® determines the percentage of moisture present in the wool sample. A small portion of wool sample was taken, with the help of a brush the fibers were parallelized, placed inside special cartridges and introduced into the equipment, which determined the moisture percentage corresponding to each sample.

Percentage of wool/hair

A small portion of wool is taken from each sample, approximately 10 fibers, then they are placed in slides in the Microscope with the 10x objective, where the structures are observed to differentiate between wool and hair fibers, and in the same way, each sample is counted.

BIBLIOGRAPHIC REFERENCES

Aguilar, F. L. 2007. Main Wool Sheep Breeds in Mexico. Licentiate Thesis.

Alvarado, P. I. 2018. Introduction to Sheep Production. Faculty of Veterinary Sciences. UNCPBA. Pp 6-16.

Alata, V. V., Ccaccya, P. I., Loayza, H. S. H., Sánchez, Ñ. O. A., Gamarra, N. W. and Huamán, C. L. 2000. Washing method for alpaca fleece. Micaela Bastidas National University of Apurimac. 3,4.

Andrade, M. M. S. 2017. Textiles. Available at: http://ri.uaemex.mx/bitstream/handle/20.500.11799/70597/secme-29747_1.pdf?sequence=1. Accessed: February 17, 2020.

Araoz, M. R. 2019. Relationship between follicular density, fiber diameter, wick length and fleece weight in first and second shearing alpacas, in the Coarita-Paratía breeding module. Licentiate thesis. National University of the Altiplano. Faculty of Veterinary Medicine and Animal Husbandry. Peru.

Arteaga, C. J. D. 2007. Mexican Association of Sheep Breeders. AMCO. Current diagnosis of the situation of sheep in Mexico. Available at: http://www.uno.org.mx/razas_ovinas/catalogo_razas.pdf. Accessed: October 2018.

Arrebola, M.F. 2002. Genetic characterization of the wool aptitude of the Spanish native merino. Available at: https://helvia.uco.es/xmlui/bitstream/handle/10396/301/13208378.pdf?sequence=1&isAllowed=y. Accessed: February 11, 2020.

Arrebola, M. F. A., Varela, C. M., & Molina A. A. (2004). Genetic characterization of the wool aptitude of the Spanish native merino. Available at: https://www.juntadeandalucia.es/export/drupaljda/1337165058lana_merino.pdf. Accessed: February 12, 2020.

Atto, M. J. A. 2007. Importance of tropical sheep introduced to the country: Productive and reproductive characteristics. Arch. Latinoam. Prod. Anim. Vol. 15 (Suppl. 1).

AWI. 2004. Australian Wool Innovation. Pricemaker. http://www.pricemaker.info/index.html.

Badajoz, L. E. 2007. Determination of alpaca fiber fineness associated with the secondary follicle/primary follicle (S/P) ratio between Suri and Huacaya breeds. Licentiate Thesis. Universidad Nacional Mayor de San Marcos. Faculty of Veterinary Medicine. Lima, Peru

Bancks, R. G and Brown, D. J. 2009. Genetic improvement in the Australasian Merino management of a diverse gene pool for changing markets. Animal Genetic Resources Information. 45, 29-36. Food and Agriculture Organization of the United Nations.

Borges, I. and Gonçalves, L. C. 2002. Manual prático de caprino e ovinocultura. *Federal University of Minas Gerais, Belo Horizonte.*

Botha, A. F. and Hunter, L. 2010. The measurement of wool fibre properties and their effect on worsted processing performance and product quality. Part 1: The objective measurement of wool fibre properties. *Textile Progress*, *42*(4), 227-339.

Bustinza, V. 2001. The alpaca, knowledge of great Andean potential. Volumes I and II. Office of Learning Resources. UNA. Puno, Peru.

Carrera, C. J. M. and Benjamín, C. C. 2011. Characteristics of Sheep Production in the Municipality of Pinos, Zacatecas: the Municipality with the Largest National Sheep Inventory. Autonomous University of Ciudad Juarez, Chihuahua. University Texts Collection, Research Series. Vol. 1.

Cazares, R. R. E. 2008. Optimization of the Dyeing and Finishing Process of Polyester/Wool Fabrics with Forosyn Dyes. Bachelor's Thesis. Technical University of the North. School of Engineering in Applied Sciences. School of Textile Engineering. Ibarra, Ecuador.

Cortada, M. M. 2011. Dynamics of project formulation: Merino wool case. Doctoral dissertation, University of Buenos Aires. Available at: https://core.ac.uk/download/pdf/144233157.pdf. Accessed: February 10, 2020.

Chancusig, P. S. A. 2011. Sheep Skin Tanning with the Use of Different Levels of Tanal W for Carpet Production (Bachelor's thesis).

Costa, R. G., Jacinto, M. A. C., Camacho, M. E., Medeiros, A. N., Oliveira, R. J. F. and Rey, S. 2006. Structural aspects of sheep skin and its resistance. Sitio Argentino de Producción Animal. pR 7, no. 2: 24-29.

Delgado, S. D. J. 2003. Perspectives of Llama Fiber Production in Bolivia. Potential and development of strategies to improve fiber quality and marketability (Doctoral dissertation, PhD thesis, Hohenheim University, Germany). Pp 3-7

Deurden, J. E. J. Text. Inst. 20 (1929) pp. T93-T100.

Elvira, M. G. 2009. Sheep: the biological wool factory. *Technical information folder. Livestock. EEA Esquel*, (32).

Espinal, C. F., Martínez, C. H., and Amézquita, V. J. E. 2006. The sheep and goat chain in Colombia. Available at: http://bibliotecadigital.agronet.gov.co/bitstream/11348/3914/1/20078611357_caracterizacion_ovinosycaprinos.pdf. Accessed: December 4, 2019.

Falconí, H. A. J. 2013. Improvement Proposal to Increase the Yield in the Sheep Wool Production Process in a Textile Company by Changing the Preparation and Dosage of the Ensimaje. Bachelor's Thesis. Industrial Engineering. Santa Maria Catholic University. Arequipa, Peru.

FAO [1]. 2009. The International Year OF Natural Fibres. Available at: https://studylib.es/doc/5064614/45-2009---food-and-agriculture-organization-of-the-united.... Accessed: November 25, 2019. FAO [2]. 2009. Sheep and Goats for diverse products and profits. Available at: http://www.fao.org/3/a-i0524e.pdf%20pagina%209. Accessed: December 5, 2019.

FAO[1]. 2020. Meat and meat products, Available at: http://www.fao.org/ag/againfo/themes/es/meat/home.html. Accessed: January 2020.

FAO[2]. 2020. Sheep. Available at: http://www.fao.org/livestock-systems/global-distributions/sheep/en/. Accessed: January 2020.

FAOSTAT[1]. 2020. World Sheep Population. Available at: http://www.fao.org/faostat/en/#data/QA. Accessed: January 2020.

FAOSTAT[2]. 2020. Wool production. Available at: http://www.fao.org/faostat/es/#data/QL. Accessed: January 2020.

Fernández-d'Arlas, B., Peña, R. C., and Eceiza, A. 2016. Extraction of keratin from "Latxa" sheep wool. *Revista Iberoamericana de Polímeros*, *17*(3), 110-121.

Frey, A., Martín, N., De Caro, A., Álvarez Ugarte, D. and Elvira, M. 2005. Variation of Average Fiber Diameter in Merino Sheep Translocated from Patagonia to the Pampas Region in Argentina. Available at: https://www.agro.uba.ar/sites/default/files/catedras/variacion_diametro_promedio_fibras_ovejas_meri.pdf. Accessed: May 2020.

Frey, A. 2007. Wool quality in Argentina. Available at: https://www.agro.uba.ar/sites/default/files/catedras/calidad_lanas_argentina.pdf. Accessed: February 20, 2020.

Galicer, J. A. 2015. Sheep. University of Belgrano. Faculty of Agricultural Sciences. Buenos Aires, Argentina.

Ganzábal, A. 2014. Guía Práctica de Producción Ovina en Pequeña Escala en Iberoamérica. Available at: https://citarea.cita-aragon.es/citarea/bitstream/10532/2714/1/2014_295.pdf Accessed: February 6, 2020.

García V. W. and Sota C. W. 2007. Effect of fineness on fiber production and live weight gain at different animal ages and at contracting times of the year. APPA -ALPA -Cusco, Peru.

Germano, C. R., Méndez, S. A., Freitas, O. R. J., Camacho, E., Rey, S., Vallecillo, A. and Delgado, B. J. V. 2006. Histological characterization of the skin of kids of the Blanca Serrana Andaluza breed. Available at: https://helvia.uco.es/bitstream/handle/10396/6289/feagas29-2006.1-2.pdf?sequence=1. Accessed: February 2020.

Gómez, M. B. (2017). *Characterization of the wool and productive potential of sheep biotypes present in the Central Region of Argentina* (Doctoral dissertation, Catholic University of Córdoba).

Grossman, B. 2009. Study of the Textile Sector in Bolivia. United Nations Industrial Development Organization, La Paz, Bolivia, 15-27.

Guzmán, B. J. C. 2009. Evaluation of the Corriedale Sheep (*Ovis aries*) Fleece Grading Method at S.A.I.S. Pachacutec. Master Thesis. Molina National Agrarian University. Post Graduate School of Animal Production. Lima, Peru.

Hernández, M. J. A., Valencia, P. M., Ruíz, N. J. E. Mireles, A. A. I., Cortez, R. C. and Gallegos, S. J. 2017. Contribution of Oviniculture to the Livestock Sector in Mexico. Agroproductividad. Vol. 10 Issue 3, p87-93. 7p.

Huanca, T., Apaza, N. and Lazo, A. 2007. Evaluation of fiber diameter in alpacas from the communities of the districts of Cojata and Santa Rosa Puno. APPA - ALPA -Cusco, Peru.

INEGI. 2007. General Description of Sheep. El Ganado Ovino en México, Censo Agropecuario 2007-2013. SNIEG. Available at: http://internet.contenidos.inegi.org.mx/contenidos/productos/prod_serv/contenidos/espanol/bvinegi/productos/censos/agropecuario/2007/ganderia/ovino/mex/GanovinMex3.pdf. Accessed: October 15, 2018.

INEGI. 2007. Total sheep stock by activity and zootechnical function. Available at: https://www.inegi.org.mx/contenidos/programas/cagf/2007/tabulados/Tabulado_Mpio_VIII_CAGyF_64.pdf. Accessed: November 28, 2019.

Khan, M. J., Abbas, A., Ayaz, M., Naeem, M., Saleem, A. M. and Hussain, S. M. 2012. Factors affecting wool quality and quantity in sheep. African Journal of Biotechnology Vol. 11(73), pp. 13761-13766.

Lewer, R. P., Woolaston, R. R., & Howe, R. R. (1994). Studies on Western Australian Merino Sheep. II. Genetic and phenotypic parameter estimates for objectively measured traits on ram and ewe hoggets using different model types. *Australian Journal of Agricultural Research*, *45*(4), 829-840.

Lockuán, L. F. E. 2013. The textile industry and its quality control. Textile Fibers. Available at: https://books.google.es/books?hl=en&lr=&id=al9HRXxdx6kC&oi=fnd&pg=PA2&dq=classification%C3%B3n+of+the+textile+fibers&ots=6JUyO8ATtn&sig=F5_ofWXT6lMJietpuDlfHZwbAVw#v=onepage&q=classification%C3%B3n%20of%20fibers%20textiles&f=false. Accessed November 27, 2019.

Lujan, M. M. A. and Hernández, B. M. 2018. Effect of sex and age on wool characteristics of Rambouillet sheep in a semi-intensive system in Zacatecas. Bachelor's thesis. Autonomous University of Zacatecas "Francisco García Salinas". Academic Unit of Veterinary Medicine and Animal Husbandry. Zacatecas, Mexico.

Lupton, C. J., McColl, A. and StobarT, R. H. 2006. Fiber characteristics of the Huacaya Alpaca. Small Ruminant Research. 64. 211-224pp.

Marín, C. V., and Monroy, B. G. 2013. SUSTAINABLE NATURAL TEXTILE FIBERS AND NEW CONSUMPTION HABITS. Legado de Arquitectura y Diseño Magazine, (13), 31-45.

Mario, G. E. 2015. Wool: Global and Domestic Market, Prospects and Quality. Available at: https://inta.gob.ar/sites/default/files/script-tmp-inta_lanas_mercado_mundial_nacional_2015.pdf. Accessed: December 10, 2019.

Martínez, M. E., de la Barra, R., Ortega, I. L., Pavez, P., Guarda, P., Suazo, C. P. and Díaz, I. 2018. Technification of the artisanal conditioning and transformation process of pigmented sheep wool and hides in the Los Lagos Region.

Molina, F. 2013. Sheep. Available at: http://www.produccion-animal.com.ar/produccion_ovina/produccion_ovina/000-ganado_lanar_en_argentina_libro/06-capitulo_2.pdf. Accessed: October 23, 2018.

Montes, M., Quicaño, I., Quispe, R., Quispe, E. C. and Alfonso, L. 2008. Quality characteristics of Huacaya Alpaca fibre produced in the Peruvian Andean Plateau region of Huancavelica. Span. J. of Agric. Res. 6(1):33-38pp.

Mueller, J. 1999. Superfine wool production. National Institute of Agricultural Technology, EEA Bariloche.

Mueller, J.P., Bidinost, F. and Taddeo, H.R. 2003. Genetic Parameters in Two Patagonian Merino Cattle. RIA, 32 (3): 161-172. INTA, Argentina.

Mueller, J., Sacchero, D., and Duga, L. 2005. Genotype-environment interaction on the production of superfine wool sheep in Patagonia. Wool quality. Revista Argentina de Producción Animal, 25(3-4), 143-152.

Mueller, J. P and Cueto, M. I. 2010. Strategies of the wool sector to improve and increase its use among textile fibers. Memorias. Available at: https://inta.gob.ar/sites/default/files/script-tmp-inta-manual_actualizacion_en_produccion_ovina.pdf#page=149. Accessed: February 17, 2020.

Orona, C. I., López, M. J., Vázquez, V. C., Salazar, S. E. and Ramírez, R. M. 2014. Microeconomic Analysis of a Representative Sheep Meat Production Unit in the State of Mexico Under a Semi Intensive Production System. Revista Mexicana de Agronegocios, vol. 34. pp 720-728.

Pacsi, C. G. L. 2016. "Effect of Chirca Blanca (*Baccharis dracunculifolia*) Extract in the Tanning Process Sheep Skin (*Ovis orientalis aries*) and Alpaca Skin (*Vicugna pacos*) for Obtaining Wet- White Hides". Licentiate Thesis. National University of the Altiplano. Faculty of Agrarian Sciences. Professional School of Agroindustrial Engineering.

Peña, S. 2019. Genetic and morphological characterization of criollo sheep from Argentina. Doctoral dissertation, Universidad Nacional de La Plata.

Peña, S., López, G., Abiatti, N. and Martínes, R. D. 2017. Wool fineness characteristics of sheep breeds in Argentina. Revista de Divulgación Técnica Agropecuaria, Agroindustrial y Ambiental. Faculty of Agricultural Sciences. UNLZ. Vol. 4 (4): 35-45.

Pesok, M. J. C. 2015. Wool. Composition, Structure and Properties. Available at: https://sites.google.com/site/introtecnotextil/iii---la-lana-composicion-estructura-y-propiedades. Accessed: February 14, 2020.

Poma, G. A. G. and Ventura, C. A. E. 2009. Characterization of the fiber diameter profile in white Huacaya alpacas. Licentiate Thesis. National University of Huancavelica. Faculty of Engineering Sciences. Academic Professional School of Animal Husbandry. Huancavelica, Peru.

Quispe, P. E., Poma, G. A. and Purroy, U. A. 2013. Productive and textile characteristics of huacaya breed alpaca fiber. Computense Journal of Veterinary Sciences. 7(1) 1-29.

Reveles, V. C. 2018. Characterization of Dorper Sheep Fibers in an Intensive System in Central Zacatecas.

Bachelor's Thesis. Autonomous University of Zacatecas "Francisco García Salinas". Academic Unit of Veterinary Medicine and Animal Husbandry. Zacatecas, Mexico.

Romero, M. J. 2005. Background of Oviniculture in Mexico. Unit 4. Sheep husbandry. Autonomous University of Chihuahua. Pp 139-169.

Rosas, R. R. A. 2016. Sheep Wool as an Insulating Material: natural, renewable and sustainable. Master's Thesis. Building Engineering. Polytechnic University of Catalonia.

Sacchero, D. M., and Mueller, J. P. 2007. Differences in Fiber Diameter Profile, Strand Length, and Wool Tensile Strength in selected and unselected Merino Herds. RIA. Revista de Investigaciones Agropecuarias, 36(2), 49-61. INTA, Argentina.

Sacchero, D. 2012. Fiber Diameter Profiles in prepartum wools of Merino sheep. Available at: https://www.researchgate.net/publication/279537459_Perfiles_de_Diametro_de_Fibra_en_lanas_preparto_de_ovejas_Merino/link/55967e2308ae793d137b7890/download. Accessed: May 2020.

Sánchez, B. A. L. 2010. Study of genetic associations between pigmentation traits and wool production and quality traits in the Corriedale breed. Available at: https://kipdf.com/estudio-de-las-asociaciones-geneticas-entre-caracteristicas-de-pigmentacion-y-ca_5ae8091d7f8b9a15838b45a2.html. Accessed: May 2020.

Sandoval, G. N. C. 2019. Evaluation of carcass and meat quality of five sheep breeds under the same management. Available at: https://bdigital.zamorano.edu/bitstream/11036/6509/1/AGI-2019-T055.pdf. Accessed: February 2020.

SAGARPA. 2015. Propuesta de capacitación para el desarrollo de capacidades pecuarias con visión empresarial orientadas a micro, pequeños y medianos productores de ganado ovino. Available at: https://www.gob.mx/cms/uploads/attachment/file/346968/Capacidad_Pecuaria_Detallado.pdf. Accessed: February 6, 2020.

SAGARPA. 2016. Plan Rector Sistema Productivo Ovinos (2015-2024) Available at: http://spo.uno.org.mx/wp-content/uploads/2016/05/plan_rector_ovinos2016.pdf.pdf. Accessed: December 11, 2019.

SAGARPA. 2017. Oviniculture, a very tucking activity. Available at: https://www.gob.mx/agricultura/es/articulos/la-ovinocultura-una-actividad-muy-arropadora. Accessed: December 11, 2019.

Saldaña, P. L. N. 2017. Categorization, classification and industrial processing of alpaca fiber. Bachelor's thesis. Universidad Nacional Agraria la Molina. Faculty of Animal Husbandry. Lima, Perú.

SIAP[1]. 2018. Livestock production advance by state. Available at: http://infosiap.siap.gob.mx/repoAvance_siap_gb/pecAvanceEdo.jsp. Accessed: December 4, 2019.

SIAP[2]. 2018. Livestock production advance by product. Available at: http://infosiap.siap.gob.mx/repoAvance_siap_gb/pecAvanceProd.jsp. Accessed: December 4, 2019.

SIAP[3]. 2018. Open data. Livestock production statistics 2018. Available at: http://infosiap.siap.gob.mx/gobmx/datosAbiertos_p.php. Accessed: November 28, 2019.

SIAP[4]. 2018. A Visit to the 2017 Agrifood Atlas, Wool: another face of sheep. Available at: https://www.gob.mx/siap/articulos/una-visita-al-atlas-agroalimentario-2017-la-lana-otra-cara-del-ovino?idiom=es. Accessed: February 15, 2020.

SIAP. 2020. Statistical yearbook of livestock production. Wool Available at: https://nube.siap.gob.mx/cierre_pecuario/. Accessed: January 2020.

SIAP. 2019. Dirty wool. Monthly livestock production advance. Available at: http://infosiap.siap.gob.mx/repoAvance_siap_gb/pecAvanceProd.jsp. Accessed: December 11, 2019.

SIAP-SAGARPA. 2018. Livestock population 2008-2017, Sheep, Heads. Available at: https://www.gob.mx/cms/uploads/attachment/file/412568/Ovino__2017.pdf. Accessed: November 28, 2019.

Solis, R. 2000. Second Edition "Production of South American Camelids" Second Edition. 550p.

SPH. 2015. Wool Chapter from the Sheep Production Handbook. American Sheep Industry Association, Inc. 2015 Edition. Vol. 8.

Suárez, V. 2004. Sheep Dairy and Pampinta Breed. IDIA XXI-Sheep,4(7), 194-200.

Taipe, L. C. 2012. Evaluation of three levels of metal complex in the dyeing process in sheep (*Ovis aries)* leather. Licentiate Thesis. National University of Huancavelica. Faculty of Agricultural Sciences. Acobamba, Huancavelica.

Tinoco, G. O. 2009. Sheep wool production chain in the textile and apparel sector. *Industrial data, 12(*2), 73-80.

Toapanta, Y. A. M. 2016. Morphological evaluation of wool fiber from sheep at CEYPSA. Undergraduate Thesis. Veterinary Medicine. Technical University of Cotopaxi. Academic Unit of Agricultural Sciences and Natural Resources.

Villegas, M. C. and González, M. B. 2013. Sustainable natural textile fibers and new consumption habits. Available at: http://ri.uaemex.mx/bitstream/handle/20.500.11799/79555/03.pdf?sequence=1. Accessed: November 25, 2019.

Zenteno, H. E. J. 2015. Textile in the interior space (Bachelor's thesis, Universidad del Azuay).

Zúñiga, R. J. A. 2013. Evaluation of three Chromium Sulfate Levels in Aniline Binding for Dyeing Sheep Wool (Bachelor's thesis).

Kolibri 360 GmbH
Ferdinand-Jühlke-Straße 7
99095 Erfurt, Deutschland
produktsicherheit@kolibri360.de

Druck:
CPI Druckdienstleistungen GmbH
im Auftrag der
Kolibri 360 GmbH
Ferdinand-Jühlke-Str. 7
99095 Erfurt